INTERMITTENT FASTING DIET PLAN

The step-by-step guide to boost metabolism healthy weight loss, detox your body with diet plan and intermittent fasting.

3 BOOK OF 12

By David Johnson

Chapter 1. Intermittent Fasting Diet Plan and Metabolic Health

In the course of the last 10 to 15 years, intermittent fasting has arisen as an unpredictable way to deal with lessen body weight and improve metabolic wellbeing past basic calorie limitation. In this audit, we sum up discoveries identified with Ramadan and Sunnah fasting. We at that point talk about the part of caloric limitation as an intercession for weight control, yet critically, as a procedure for solid maturing and life span. At long last, we audit the four most normal intermittent fasting (IF) procedures used to date for weight the board and to improve cardio metabolic wellbeing. Weight reduction is regular after intermittent fasting yet doesn't have all the earmarks of being not quite the same as day by day caloric limitation when thought about straightforwardly. On the off chance that may likewise give extra cardio metabolic advantage, like insulin refinement, that is free from weight reduction. While no particular fasting routine stands apart as unrivaled as of now, there is for sure heterogeneity in reactions to these unique intermittent fasting eats less. This recommends that one dietary routine may not be obviously appropriate for each person. Future examinations ought to think about procedures for fitting dietary remedies, including intermittent fasting, in light of cutting edge phenotyping and genotyping before diet commencement.

powerful methods, for example, the hyperinsulinemic euglycemic clip, are justified to additional logical comprehension of the impact of Ramadan fasting on metabolic wellbeing.

1.3.2 Sunnah Fasting

Sunnah fasting is rehearsed year round and remembers fasting week after week for Mondays and Thursdays with an extra 6 days of fasting in the Shawwal month. Two examinations by a similar exploration bunch surveyed 12 weeks of week after week Sunnah fasting joined with every day CR in more established guys from Malaysia. Sunnah fasting comprised of a little dinner preceding dawn and a full supper after nightfall; also, members were approached to limit calories by 300 to 500 kcal/d and to build admission of good food varieties. The two investigations demonstrated a general energy shortfall of 18% and weight reduction of 3%. Fat mass diminished by about 6% to 8%. While fat free mass was unaltered in one examination, another investigation showed a slight reduction that was not fundamentally not quite the same as the benchmark group. Just surveyed cardio metabolic results and noted reductions in both absolute cholesterol and LDL cholesterol by 8% and a diminishing in systolic and diastolic blood pressures by 4.5% and 2.6%, separately. There was no adjustment of glucose, and insulin was not announced.

Extra work by looked at whether as an accentuation on faith based dietary practices could advance wellbeing following Ramadan for 12 weeks. The benchmark group was relegated to standard dietary counsel, while the mediation bunch was additionally given faith based dietary guidance, for example, the incorporation of Sunnah fasting. The event of fasting twice week by week (Monday and Thursday) was unaltered; nonetheless, fasting once week by week (Monday or Thursday) expanded in the mediation bunch. There was no adjustment of fasting recurrence in the benchmark group. A decline in BMI from standard was seen in the mediation bunch, yet was not altogether unique in relation to the benchmark group. The mediation bunch likewise experienced humble upgrades in cardio metabolic wellbeing, for example, diminishes in diastolic circulatory strain and expansions in HDL cholesterol. Notwithstanding, this could likewise be a result of upgraded vegetable admission happening in the mediation bunch. Together, these examinations recommend that the act of Sunnah fasting may advance cardio metabolic wellbeing. A continuation of Ismail et al. on a bigger and more generalizable scale could have general wellbeing suggestions inside Muslim people group.

1.4 Intermittent Fasting improve Weight Management

In this segment, we survey the extraordinary IF procedures that have been read for weight the board, with included accentuation their cardio metabolic wellbeing sway. These incorporate the 5:2 eating regimen, ADF, ADMF, and TRF.

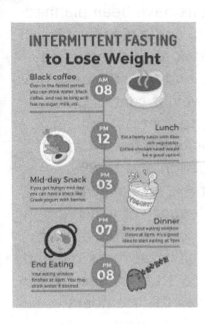

1.4.1 The 5:2 Intermittent Fasting Diet Plan

The 5:2 eating routine is a mainstream diet that imparts a few similitudes to Sunnah fasting, as the two regimens call for altered fasting to happen twice week after week. Until now, all 5:2 regimens have permitted 25% energy admission on the "quick day" as opposed to a total quick. This taking care of routine, joined with not obligatory benefiting from the excess 5 days, may inspire a week by week energy deficiency of 20 to 25%. Dinners devoured during the changed quick days are commonly eaten whenever. About portion of the preliminaries license members to choose two no consecutive quick days, while others require a more forceful methodology with back to back quick days.

Weight, body shape, appetite, and energy consumption changes

All 5:2 eating routine examinations have been planned as weight reduction intercessions, and a significant number of these investigations look at 5:2 versus day by day CR. Short term examines enduring 8 weeks have revealed high adherence to 5:2 weight control plans. In general adherence doesn't seem to contrast among 5:2 and day by day CR. Intercessions going from 4 to 24 weeks have detailed weight reduction of 4 to 8%. Weight reduction of in any event 5% is conceivable inside about two months. The adequacy of achieving in any event 5% weight reduction is comparable among 5:2 and day by day CR. Diminishes in fat mass regularly range from 9 to 13% with simply a 1 to 4% decrease in fat free mass and is like day by day CR. Members likewise report lower caloric admission during 5:2 contrasted with day by day CR. Diminished admission could be the consequence of transient ketosis, which may incompletely clarify the noticed concealment of craving evaluations and support of gauge ghrelin focus during 5:2 a chemical which generally increments with weight reduction and signs hunger. Introductory evaluations of yearning are higher during 5:2 contrasted with day by day CR yet seem, by all accounts, to be relieved by higher protein allow and standardize after some time. Further examination ought to interpret feed and quick day collaborations on yearning, totality, and satiation, while matching insights with biomarkers of craving.

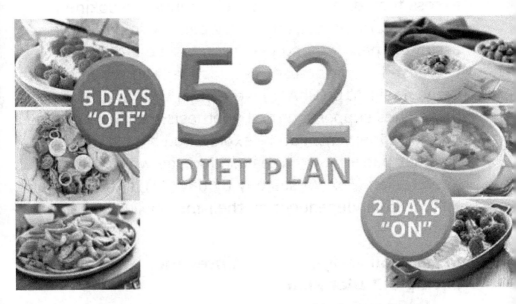

5:2 DIET PLAN
5 DAYS "OFF"
2 DAYS "ON"

Cardio metabolic health changes during 5:2 Diet Plan

Comparative weight reduction results make it conceivable to analyze weight loss independent cardio metabolic contrasts among 5:2 and day by day CR. Diminishes in absolute cholesterol, LDL cholesterol, and fatty substances as high as 13%, 15%, and 22%, separately, have been accounted for with 5:2. Humble upgrades in lipids are comparable among 5:2 and every day CR. The 5:2 eating regimen, in any case, seems to have an unrivaled insulin sensitizing sway. First noticed enhancements in insulin affectability following a half year of 5:2, which was marginally better compared to every day CR. Comparable discoveries were duplicated in two different examinations from similar agents. These perceptions could be clarified by the emotional expansion in insulin affectability quickly following 2 days of back to back fasting that waited all through the excess feed days. Moreover, differential adipokine reactions among 5:2 and every day CR could likewise assume a part. Among people with type 2 diabetes, decreased medicine use (i.e., insulin) and brought down hemoglobin A1C (HbA1c) were seen with 5:2, along these lines supporting the hypothesis that 5:2 advances insulin refinement. Future exploration should address whether pattern attributes can foresee which dietary intercession (5:2 versus day by day CR) is the best for an individual dependent on their metabolic wellbeing status.

Studies on weight loss maintenance and follow up during 5:2 Diet Plan

Following fruition of a 5:2 eating regimen, weight recapture is exceptionally factor and like day by day CR. Announced a 33% weight recover in returning members upon a 2 year follow up. In a similar report, HbA1c expanded, while complete cholesterol and LDL cholesterol got back to standard. Critically, different investigations diminished weight recapture while keeping up decreases in adiposity and cardio metabolic illness hazard through proceeded with commitment in weight reduction upkeep programs enduring 4 to 24 weeks. In examinations lacking kept advising, weight recapture happened and cardio metabolic hazard bounced back during follow ups enduring roughly a half year.

1.5 Alternate Day Modified Fasting and Alternate Day Fasting

Both ADF and ADMF switch back and forth between long periods of fasting and taking care of. Fasting days can go from 75 to 100% CR relying upon the fasting routine, and taking care of days are generally not obligatory. Fundamental work in this field used either a total quick (ADF) or a 20 hour quick every other day (ADMF). The inclusive daytime fasting has been concentrated less as often as possible because of helpless decency of a total quick every other day. Therefore, most ADMF conventions currently incorporate a solitary early afternoon dinner, which commonly falls inside a 2 hour taking care of window and allots 25% of energy prerequisites.

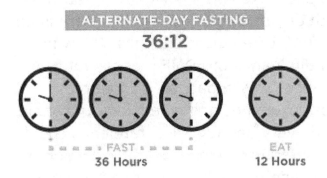

ALTERNATE-DAY FASTING
36:12

FAST
36 Hours

EAT
12 Hours

Changes in body composition, appetite and body weight during Alternate day fasting

ADF and ADMF preliminaries in people frequently bring about weight reduction either by plan or inadvertently, which is rather than mouse models exhibiting weight upkeep. Three short term preliminaries in male members were fruitful at keeping up body weight. Different preliminaries urged members to devour 145 to 200% of their energy needs on the feed days, yet members actually experienced accidental weight reduction. These reports recommend that ADF and

ADMF regimens may have helpful worth as heftiness medicines. Mediations enduring 4 to about four months report weight reduction between 3 to 13%, while preliminaries stretching out to 24 weeks report weight reduction of 6 to 11%. Correlations of day by day CR against ADF and ADMF exhibit practically identical reductions in body weight and fat mass. Some of which report patterns for more noteworthy weight reduction during ADF or ADMF. Different irregularities exist. For instance, ADMF beat every day CR for weight reduction for the initial 4 months, yet not at ensuing time points reaching out to a half year. In different cases, ADMF inspired prevalent decreases in weight and fat mass contrasted with day by day CR. Similarly, there is no agreement as for fat free mass changes. A few no randomized preliminaries of ADMF propose fat free mass maintenance. This impact on fat free mass isn't rehashed across examines and is regularly the same contrasted with every day CR. Disparate ends could originate from differing levels of weight reduction, span of intercessions, and errors between body structure evaluation strategies (i.e., bioelectrical impedance versus dual energy X ray absorptiometry).

In spite of by and large high dietary adherence, for the most part great examination maintenance, and insignificant announced results, a few ADF or ADMF considers have detailed dropout rates more prominent than 20%. True to form, dropouts expanded when the span of the intercession was 12 weeks or more. It likewise stays muddled how well tolerated these kinds of IF eats less really are contrasted with every day CR, little examinations (20 members for every gathering) seem to report comparative dropout rates, while, bigger investigations (40 members) are ambiguous. These discoveries combined with inborn individual inconstancy in noticed weight reduction and the developing interest for exact clinical treatment, recommend that individualized weight reduction approaches might be advantageous. On the side of this, identification as a "major eater" was adversely connected with weight reduction probably because of the capacity to all the more likely make up for the quick day energy deficiency. There additionally gives off an impression of being differential reactions among segment bunches after pooling a few ADMF concentrates in an auxiliary investigation. Caucasians and more seasoned people experienced bigger weight reduction, which is steady with other day by day CR contemplates. Explanations behind these distinctions stay obscure, however both social and physiological underpinnings likely assume a part.

A group has investigated a few ADMF varieties that could expand worthiness and adherence. The standard ADMF approach takes into consideration just a solitary early afternoon dinner to be devoured on fasting days. Regularly, a low fat dietary example is suggested or given. This might be hard for calorie counters liking to eat later in the day or those wanting higher fat suppers. Inspected dinner timing and recurrence during ADMF and noticed no impact regarding weight reduction or changes in body organization when the quick day supper was given at various occasions or split into three little suppers. Furthermore, furnishing members with high fat suppers during ADMF likewise didn't prevent weight reduction. Other ADMF varieties have thought about whether weight reduction might be improved by fusing stimulating practices, like devouring higher dietary protein or including exercise. It is noticed that fat free mass maintenance from gauge with a high protein diet. Another investigation exhibited comparable decreases in body weight, fat mass, fat free mass, and instinctive adiposity between high protein varieties of ADMF and every day CR. Neither examination straightforwardly contrasted a high protein ADMF approach with a standard ADMF approach. There have been immediate correlations among ADMF and ADMF with work out. It is accounted for that the consideration of activity expanded weight and fat mass misfortune contrasted with ADMF alone. Essentially, detailed enhancements from gauge in body weight and body creation in both ADMF and ADMF with practice conditions, yet just the practicing ADMF bunch accomplished measurably higher fat mass misfortune from the control. Curiously, practice during ADMF seems to weaken dropout rates. This assortment of work assessing dietary and exercise varieties during ADMF focuses to the capacity to tailor ADMF as per singular inclinations and weight reduction objectives.

Hunger, which is generally an exploratory result, seems, by all accounts, to be controlled and may clarify the diminished reported caloric admission on feed days. Just one investigation contrasted hunger during ADMF with every day CR and announced no distinction between the eating regimens. Appetitive reactions to ADF or ADMF fluctuate by study and evaluation strategy. Three weeks of ADF improved day by day sensations of completion; yet, hunger remained. With ADMF, hunger sensations seem to die down after just fourteen days. This demonstrates that decency might be upgraded with the consideration of a little quick day feast contrasted and a total quick, yet this examination has not been made tentatively. Diminished sensations of appetite and expanded sensations of totality have likewise been seen after longer openness to ADF and ADMF intercessions (as long as 10 weeks). This proposes craving standardization with time. Reactions to normalized supper tests, addressing physiological hunger, have been conflicting across examines. It is accounted for no adjustment of ghrelin following 3 weeks of ADF. Then again, hunger was unaltered after 8 to 12 weeks of ADMF and a slight expansion in ghrelin was noticed. Discoveries identified with totality and peptide YY (PYY), a gut peptide which signals completion, are uncertain too. It noticed a moderate expansion in PYY (16%) combined with expanded sensations of totality (10%) after ADMF, yet it showed no adjustment of PYY or completion. ADMF and ADF may, accordingly, appease hunger over the long haul, yet the systems clarifying are muddled and conflicting.

Changes in cardio metabolic health during Alternate day fasting

ADF and ADMF effect by and large cardio metabolic wellbeing, however conflict exists when looking at explicit results. For instance, fasting glucose has been appeared to both increment (5%) and decline (2 to 5%) during ADMF while others show no adjustment of preliminaries enduring at any rate a month and a half.

Moreover, fasting insulin may diminish 21 to 42% in examinations enduring 8 to 24 weeks, subsequently improving insulin opposition. Insulin affectability, then again, is unaltered when evaluated by means of intravenous glucose resilience test (IVGTT) and shows differential reactions to blended dinner resistance testing by sex. Because of a hyperinsuliemic euglycemic brace following two months of ADMF or day by day CR, detailed no distinction in insulin affectability. The impact of ADF on lipid focuses seems to rely upon sex and may require a more extended openness period to encounter benefits. A few examinations enduring at any rate two months have likewise shown aggregate enhancements in lipid profiles described by diminished fatty substances, LDL cholesterol, and absolute cholesterol. Advantages in all out lipid focuses are not all inclusive and may not be unique in relation to every day CR. Three investigations report no distinctions from every day CR for aggregate or LDL cholesterol after weight reduction, while another focuses to body weight free enhancements preferring ADMF. Critically, the improvement in the atherosclerotic profile of lipid particles appears to reliably improve, and introductory discoveries recommend it might beat day by day CR.

Reaction as per metabolic wellbeing status is maybe really convincing. A clinical preliminary in members with metabolic condition showed a more prominent diminishing in fasting glucose after ADMF contrasted with day by day CR, however no distinction in insulin opposition or fasting insulin focuses were noticed. Other auxiliary examinations give fundamental proof that ADMF might be more compelling than day by day CR for lessening diabetes hazard. Members with the most significant level of insulin opposition encountered the best improvement after ADMF. In an alternate examination of just insulin safe members, there were checked lessening after ADMF contrasted with day by day CR for fasting insulin (52% versus 14%, separately) and insulin obstruction (53% versus 17%, individually). Long term randomized clinical preliminaries are required in populaces with diabetes or pre diabetes to make explicit determinations in regards to sickness results after ADF or ADMF.

Studies on weight loss maintenance and follow up Alternate day fasting

Weight reduction upkeep following ADF and ADMF is sketchy. Until now, four examinations have assessed weight reduction upkeep all utilizing incomprehensibly various methodologies. Following two months of ADF or day by day CR, detailed huge weight recapture (30% of starting misfortune) in both eating regimen bunches during a 24 week unaided follow up period. Both eating regimen bunches kept up supreme misfortunes in fat and fat free mass. The corresponding tweaks, be that as it may, in percent fat mass and percent fat free mass were better with ADF contrasted with day by day CR.

This could be because of certain members keeping up ADF during the solo follow up. In the longest weight support correlation between ADMF (half CR on the quick day) and day by day CR, announced comparable weight recapture directions between every day CR and ADMF and no distinction in body creation. Curiously, people accomplishing at any rate 5% weight reduction,

27

selected higher protein consumption all through the preliminary. Different investigations combined ADMF with day by day CR during the weight reduction stage while joining admission of higher dietary protein as a feature of the weight upkeep approach. Utilized high protein feast substitutions on feed (1000 kcal/d) and quick (600 kcal/d) days during weight reduction. During weight upkeep, a similar quick day dinner substitutions were utilized while the feed days decreased dependence on supper substitutions. Members experienced limited quantities of proceeded, yet genuinely immaterial, weight reduction (1 kg) more than 12 weeks of weight reduction upkeep. Cardio metabolic enhancements just arrived at importance after weight support, despite the fact that there was clinically huge weight reduction (5%) during the weight reduction stage. Contrasted ADMF with calorie restricted feed days with every day CR alone. Following the weight reduction stage, abstains from food similarly kept up weight reduction by following proposals for higher protein consumes less calories for an extra two months. Notwithstanding approach, way of life changes causing a supported energy shortfall are needed to accomplish effective weight reduction upkeep. Further examination is expected to decide if protein admission during ADF of ADMF impacts consistence, craving, or body arrangement.

1.6 Time Restricted Feeding

Rather than 5:2, ADF, and ADMF regimens, TRF doesn't deliberately force CR. Maybe, TRF expands the day by day fasting time frame by confining food admission to a decreased window of time. Until this point, many creature examines have revealed that TRF induces clear medical advantages, remembering decreases for body weight, food consumption, hyperlipidemia, ectopic fat, and markers of irritation, just as upgrades in heart wellbeing, malignancy results, and life expectancy expansion. Late TRF preliminaries in people have permitted a taking care of window between 4 to 12 hours, albeit a window of 10 hours is believed to be ideal dependent on glycogenolysis, unsaturated fat oxidation, and gluconeogenesis regulations happening without dietary glucose accessibility.

TIME
RESTRICTED
FEEDING

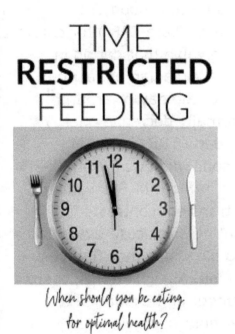

When should you be eating for optimal health?

Single arm TRF preliminaries have revealed 2 to 3% weight reduction more than 1 to 4 months. Gill and Panda enlisted 8 people with overweight and weight who detailed an eating span of more than 14 hour to pick a 10 hour not obligatory eating window of their decision for about four months. Critically, the members experienced weight reduction, diminished yearning around evening time, expanded in general energy levels, and improved rest fulfillment, which endured for 1 year after the intercession started. Another new examination enlisted more seasoned, inactive grownups with overweight and heftiness and confined their eating to 8 hour not obligatory adaptable taking care of window; study chips in likewise experienced huge weight decrease.

In more controlled preliminaries, eating prior in the day ("early TRF") or in the day ("early afternoon TRF") outflanked eating later in the day ("late TRF") for cardio metabolic wellbeing. It is conceivable that eating in synchronization with the normal circadian endocrine beat promptly in the first part of the day or around noon may hold the way to normally decrease energy consumption. In only 4 days, early TRF (8:00 AM – 2:00 PM) versus control (12 hour window: 8:00 AM – 8:00 PM) modified articulation in 6 out of 8 circadian qualities. This was joined by transient contrasts portrayed by a nighttime blunting of glucose evaluated by nonstop glucose observing alongside modified view of craving and internal heat level. Alongside this, there was a general lessening in hunger and expanded fat oxidation without affecting 24 hour energy consumption. A more drawn out 5 week hybrid preliminary in guys with overweight and pre diabetes announced that early TRF (8:00 AM – 2:00 PM) really improved insulin affectability by 24% and beta cell work by 13% when contrasted with a 12 hour energy coordinated with eating window (8:00 AM – 8:00 PM).

There were additionally noteworthy decreases in pulse and oxidative pressure (8 Isoprostanes.) Directly looked at early TRF (8:00 AM – 5:00 PM) with late TRF (12:00 PM – 9:00 PM) in 15 overweight guys in a hybrid plan. TRF diminished body weight, plasma fatty substances, and postprandial glucose levels in the two gatherings, and a reduction in fasting glucose through constant glucose checking was noticed uniquely with early TRF. Late morning TRF approaches have detailed comparable upgrades in cardio metabolic wellbeing. For instance, a randomized controlled examination found that deferring breakfast and propelling supper by 1.5 hours each (or noontime TRF) for 10 weeks diminished muscle versus fat and energy consumption in an associate of for the most part female members. Another preliminary of early afternoon TRF (8 hour window: 10:00 AM – 6:00 PM) in 23 grownups with heftiness affirmed such enhancements in cardio metabolic wellbeing, including diminished body weight, energy consumption, and systolic pulse.

A couple of studies recommend that late TRF may deteriorate cardio metabolic wellbeing. Contrasted with devouring 3 dinners/d of an EU caloric eating regimen, burning through those equivalent calories inside a solitary 4 hour evening feast (1 supper/d) expanded systolic pulse, cholesterol, hunger, early daytime fasting glucose, just as postponed insulin reaction (by means of oral glucose resilience test). Nonetheless, one 8 week randomized controlled preliminary in 34 resistance trained competitors announced that late TRF (8 hour window: 1:00 – 9:00 PM) diminished fat mass while keeping up fat free mass, muscle territory, and greatest strength when contrasted with burning through similar calories across the whole day. This preliminary additionally set off a decrease in fatty substances, testosterone, insulin like development factor 1 (IGF 1), and interleukin 1 beta without any progressions in complete cholesterol or fasting glycemic markers.

1.6.1 Diet Plans of Time Restricted Eating

Is it conceivable to improve your wellbeing not by eating less, but rather by just shaving a couple of hours off your day by day eating window? A little yet encouraging new investigation recommends that limiting eating to 10 hours per day over a three month time frame can prompt weight reduction, a decrease in stomach fat, and enhancements in many danger factors that can prompt early demise. The examination, distributed in December 2019 in Cell Metabolism, included individuals determined to have metabolic disorder, a term for a few unique conditions without a moment's delay, including hypertension, high glucose, elevated cholesterol, and abundance stomach fat.

Despite the fact that analysts didn't specify what food sources or the number of calories to devour, members ate a normal of 8.6 percent less calories throughout the span of the three month time frame, and lost 3% of their body weight and 4 percent of their stomach fat. We are amped up for these outcomes, in huge part since time confined eating can be so broadly embraced in clinical practice.

Time limited eating is only one kind of intermittent fasting. Different alternatives incorporate 5:2 fasting, where you eat typically for five days and confine calories to 500 or 600 on the two different days, and substitute day fasting, where you limit calories to around 500 each and every other day.

A specialist doesn't really require additional preparation in diet or nourishment to prescribe time confined eating to patients. It's genuinely simple to disclose and for individuals to embrace. In this investigation we permitted individuals to pick their own 10 hour window for eating, which they had the option to incorporate into their every day schedule.

To perceive what effect eating for less hours daily would have on individuals with metabolic condition, examiners selected 19 individuals: 13 men and 6 ladies. Every one of the members participated in time limited eating; there was no fake treatment bunch. Most of the members were on a statin to diminish cholesterol, a medicine to decrease circulatory strain, or both. Before the investigation started, the normal eating window for the members was over 14 hours per day.

With time limited eating, you're just permitted to devour calories during specific hours. An ordinary window of eating time could be 8, 10, or even 12 hours.

In the fourteen day time frame before the examination started, scientists had the subjects record what and when they ate in a wellbeing application that can help track day by day eating, resting, and movement designs.

One strength of the examination was the granular data on the circumstance of eating it gave. It is outstanding at gauge [before the examination began] that numerous members were 'brushing' throughout the span of the day and part of the evening, with one member eating for 17 hours in a 24 hour time frame. This is likely a typical eating design in the United States today, she adds, and it can prompt abundance calorie utilization.

Every one of the members decided to start their 10 hour window between 8 a.m. what's more, 10 a.m., and end between 6 p.m. also, 8 p.m. Based on food utilization records gathered before the investigation started, specialists inferred that the members didn't skip breakfast, yet rather deferred it for a little while. The equivalent went for supper: Rather than avoiding the dinner, individuals ate their last feast before to oblige the timetable. At the point when they weren't eating, members were urged to drink water. Utilizing the wellbeing application, every individual logged what and when they ate, just as their dozing times.

There were no unfriendly occasions detailed. After the three month preliminary, not exclusively did the patients get in shape and fat, yet their "terrible" LDL cholesterol and circulatory strain dropped as well. Glucose and insulin levels started to improve also, showing better metabolic wellbeing.

The high hazard populace that this investigation included individuals with metabolic condition with gentle class one weight makes up a huge piece of the populace in the United States. As per the most recent information, more than a third of all adults in the United States meet the metabolic syndrome criteria.

1.7 Intermittent Fasting Provide Health Benefits Independent of Weight Loss

Our survey shows that intermittent fasting approaches may give medical advantages free of weight reduction. This is in concurrence with Meta analyses showing diminished fasting insulin, in spite of no distinction in weight reduction between intermittent fasting regimens and CR. It is conceivable that one intermittent fasting routine could beat another, yet this remaining parts to be straightforwardly tried. Besides, consistence to intermittent fasting and day by day CR is frequently equivalent and shows that one may not be better than the other to accomplish a negative energy balance. Regardless, rehashed models across each kind of intermittent fasting routine do demonstrate an insulin sharpening impact happening very quickly upon diet inception. It is conceivable that this intermittent fasting impact could be interceded through circadian science as diurnal varieties in glucose, energy use, and substrate usage favor eating prior in the day and fasting around evening time.

Significantly, the heterogeneity in the reaction to various intermittent fasting techniques recommends that customized approaches will improve weight reduction and upgrade cardio metabolic wellbeing. In this way, the following period of intermittent fasting exploration should tailor dietary remedies dependent on factors identified with a person's remarkable physiology, current wellbeing status, dietary inclinations, social impacts, and constructed conditions. This new section of exploration can possibly recognize ideal contender for a specific weight reduction treatment. Progressed phenotyping and genotyping to distinguish the subatomic transducers of dietary mediations may one day give the premise to better redo care.

Present day taking care of practices incorporate eating across expanded timeframes (15 hours) with the biggest extent of calories devoured in the evening. Proof from creature models presented to intermittent fasting demonstrate a circadian resetting impact that could counterbalance chronobiological desynchrony forced by 24 hour social orders. Then again, confounded food admission during intermittent fasting may add to such desynchrony. Proceeded with assessment of intermittent fasting can possibly explain the interchange between diet, digestion, and circadian physiology. Ramadan research gives understanding into postponed intermittent fasting in people as energy admission is limited to predominately evening hours and has been appeared to diminish rest and disturb circadian musicality. However our survey focuses to upgraded cardio metabolic wellbeing with Ramadan fasting. Restricting evening energy admission during reproduced night shift appears to counterbalance a portion of the cardio metabolic brokenness noted in night shift laborers. Such discoveries place that the metabolic impact of fasting may exceed that of circadian interruption. Accordingly, using intermittent fasting as a countermeasure to known and regularly unavoidable circadian disruptors, including rest limitation, social stream slack, and night shift, is a neglected space of interventional research requiring consideration.

1.8 Intermittent Fasting Aids in the Preservation of Muscle Mass

Muscle is metabolically dynamic tissue that helps keep your metabolic rate high. This assists you with consuming more calories, even very still. Sadly, the vast majority lose both fat and muscle when they get more fit.

It's been asserted that intermittent fasting could protect bulk better compared to calorie limitation because of its impact on fat copying chemicals. Specifically, the increment in human development chemical saw during fasting could help protect bulk, regardless of whether you're getting thinner.

A 2011 audit tracked down that intermittent fasting was more successful at holding muscle during weight reduction than a customary, low calorie diet. In any case, results have been blended. A later audit discovered intermittent fasting and constant calorie limitation to effect slender weight.

One ongoing investigation discovered no distinction between the slender weight of individuals who were fasting and individuals on consistent calorie limitation following two months. Nonetheless, at 24 weeks, those in the fasting bunch had lost less slender weight. Bigger and longer investigations are expected to see whether intermittent fasting is more compelling at safeguarding slender weight.

Intermittent fasting may help diminish the measure of muscle you lose when you get more fit. Nonetheless, the examination is blended. Despite the fact that examination has shown some encouraging discoveries, the impacts of intermittent fasting on digestion are as yet being explored.

Early examination proposes that transient diets support digestion as much as 14%, and a few investigations recommend that your bulk doesn't diminish much with intermittent fasting. On the off chance that this is valid, intermittent fasting has a few significant weight reduction benefits over abstains from food dependent on constant calorie limitation. By the day's end, intermittent fasting can be a profoundly compelling weight reduction device for some individuals.

Chapter 2. Intermittent Fasting Diet Plan and Type 2 Diabetes

Type 2 Diabetes is a metabolic problem described by hyperglycemia that causes various inconveniences with critical long haul grimness and mortality. The issue is fundamentally because of insulin opposition especially in liver, skeletal muscle, and fat tissue. In this audit, we detail the hormonal components prompting the improvement of diabetes and talk about whether intermittent fasting ought to be considered as another option, no restorative treatment alternative for patients with this issue.

2.1 Introduction

Type 2 Diabetes Mellitus (DM) is a typical metabolic issue portrayed by hyperglycemia brought about by different components including hindered insulin discharge, insulin opposition, diminished glucose usage, unreasonable hepatic glucose creation, and foundational poor quality irritation. As per the CDC, diabetes influences 34.2 million individuals in the United States (10.5% of the complete populace). Diabetes is known to be answerable for the improvement of different long haul difficulties, which add to the sickness' horribleness and mortality. For example, diabetes is the main source of renal disappointment, new beginning visual impairment, and no traumatic lower limit removal in the United States. The entanglements of diabetes can be either vascular or no vascular in nature. The vascular intricacies incorporate retinopathy, macular edema, mono and polyneuropathy, autonomic brokenness, nephropathy, coronary illness, fringe vascular infection and stroke. No vascular inconveniences incorporate issues with the gastrointestinal parcel (gastroparesis), changes in skin tone, expanded danger of contaminations, waterfalls, glaucoma, periodontal sickness, and hearing misfortune. At present the objective of treatment for type 2 diabetes is based on forestalling or postponing entanglements and keeping up personal satisfaction for the patient, as depicted by an agreement report for the administration of hyperglycemia by the American Diabetes Association (ADA) and European Association for the Study of Diabetes (EASD). While it is supported that patients with type 2 diabetes participate in way of life changes including expanded active work, weight reduction, and clinical sustenance treatment, a lion's share of patients require the utilization of drugs to accomplish control of their blood glucose levels. In spite of the fact that it has been very much portrayed that type 2 diabetes is a sickness of insulin obstruction, a lot of the clinical treatments that doctors use are based around the reason of giving the patient more insulin. For example, drugs like the sulfonylureas, GLP-1 agonists, DPP-4 inhibitors, and different insulin arrangements all work by either expanding the endogenous creation of insulin or expanding the measure of exogenous insulin got. While this attempts to diminish hyperglycemia in these patients, treating an illness of insulin opposition by expanding insulin might be counterproductive, prompting the necessity of expanding measures of prescription throughout an extensive stretch of time. Indeed, an examination showed that when treating type 2 diabetics with concentrated insulin treatment to accomplish tight glycemic control, the patients all created expanded hyperinsulinemia and weight acquire over a six month period.

Intermittent Fasting and Diabetes
What do the Dietitians Say?

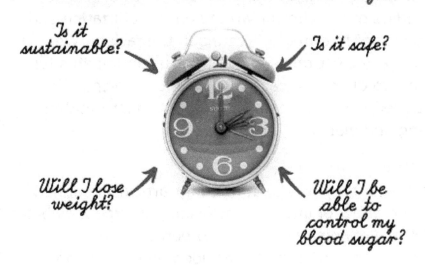

Is it sustainable?

Is it safe?

Will I lose weight?

Will I be able to control my blood sugar?

Albeit the ADA and EASD portray the objective of treatment as being pointed toward forestalling or postponing the intricacies of this infection, the objective of this audit is to investigate the chance of utilizing intermittent fasting as a no restorative alternative for the treatment of type 2 diabetes through improved insulin affectability. While thinking about the restorative job of intermittent fasting in patients with diabetes, there are three chemicals that probably assume a huge part. These incorporate insulin, just as the adipokines leptin and adiponectin. It depict the impacts of these chemicals on different tissues. It is the motivation behind this audit to give knowledge into the impact of these chemicals on the advancement of insulin obstruction and type 2 diabetes, just as the advantageous impacts of intermittent fasting on these metabolic markers. Pushing ahead, we trust this audit is an outline of the current writing on the utilization and adequacy of intermittent fasting in the facility. We additionally trust this survey fills in as an impetus for doctors to distribute case reports and participate in controlled investigations with respect to intermittent fasting and diabetes.

2.2 What Method is used?

A writing survey was performed for articles identified with the effect of intermittent fasting on type 2 diabetes mellitus. Preliminaries were incorporated if the investigation configuration included one of the three most generally announced intermittent fasting regimens: substitute day fasting, intermittent fasting, or time confined taking care of. At last, considers were incorporated if the result estimates included estimation for fasting glucose, HbA1C, fasting insulin, leptin, or adiponectin both in patients with and without a background marked by diabetes. Rejection models comprised of copies, abstracts, no English articles, articles that did exclude human subjects, those that didn't report result measures for any of the recently portrayed factors, and works that were unpublished or inconsequential to the subject of interest. Our underlying hunt returned a lot of examinations. Two analysts autonomously investigated modified works to decide if contemplates met our incorporation rules.

Studies that met measures were then additionally evaluated to decide if they would be remembered for our survey.

2.3 Intermittent Fasting and Appetite Control in Type 2 Diabetics

Intermittent fasting has as of late acquired fame as a methods for improving body arrangement and metabolic wellbeing. Intermittent fasting alludes to eating designs based around the standard of devouring next to no to no calories for time frames going from twelve hoursq to a few days with a customary example. There are a few distinct regimens of intermittent fasting. One such routine is substitute day fasting, in which long periods of fasting are isolated by long periods of not obligatory food utilization. Another technique is occasional fasting, in which people (additionally alluded to as 5:2 or 6:1 fasting). At long last, the most known strategy is time limited taking care of, in which food utilization is just permitted during a predefined window of time every day, regularly with sixteen to 20 hours day by day diets.

Heftiness is known to be a significant danger factor for the improvement of type 2 DM. There are various systems accepted to add to the advancement of insulin obstruction in corpulent patients. These incorporate, yet are not restricted to, foundational ongoing irritation and ectopic lipid affidavit. Instinctive fat tissue is referred to work as both a paracrine and endocrine organ through the emission of adipokines. These adipokines are either proinflammatory prompting persistent low level irritation, for example, leptin, or mitigating, for example, adiponectin. Leptin is known to assume a part in the guideline of body weight through motioning to the nerve center and other cerebrum districts to stifle food admission and increment energy use. The fiery impacts of leptin are likely because of its part in the creation of IL-6, which prompts the amalgamation of C-responsive protein in the liver just as up regulation of the supportive of incendiary cytokine TNF-alpha. Curiously, patients with more elevated levels of BMI and insulin opposition were found to have expanded leptin levels, potentially meaning that patients with stoutness and insulin obstruction are creating leptin obstruction too. Despite what might be expected, adiponectin is known to have antidiabetic and calming impacts. Adiponectin follows up on different receptors that outcomes in an increment in skeletal muscle and hepatic unsaturated fat oxidation, decreased hepatic gluconeogenesis, and expanded glucose take up. It additionally applies mitigating impacts through direct activity on provocative cells, activity of NF-kB, and collaborations with TNF-alpha. Adiponectin levels decline with collection of instinctive with the aim of deciding degrees of leptin and adiponectin in patients with metabolic disorder. They tracked down that in patients with the metabolic disorder, which incorporates stoutness and insulin opposition, an irregularity in degrees of leptin and adiponectin seemed to assume a part in metabolic adjustment that expanded the danger of type 2 diabetes. Strangely, a few examinations have shown that intermittent fasting, even without fat misfortune, has brought about a decrease of leptin

44

levels and an increment of adiponectin, which brings about upgrades of insulin opposition.

It has for quite some time been realized that limiting calories can lessen body weight and increment metabolic wellbeing. An investigation showed that 25% calorie decrease either through diet alone or diet related to practice prompted upgrades in insulin affectability and decrease in beta cell affectability in overweight, glucose lenient people. In any case, a few heftiness preliminaries have exhibited that people have huge trouble supporting every day calorie limitation for expanded timeframes. Then again, intermittent fasting has higher consistence and has shown guarantee in the improvement of metabolic danger factors, body arrangement, and weight reduction in fat people. It has been shown that these gainful impacts are expected to a limited extent to the shift during fasting from the use of glucose to unsaturated fats and ketones as the body's favored fuel source. During this progress the body starts to change from the combination and capacity of lipids to activation of fat as ketone bodies and free unsaturated fats. This progress of fuel source, or metabolic reinventing, has been featured as a likely component for a considerable lot of the helpful impacts of intermittent fasting. In conclusion, intermittent fasting has been appeared to diminish adiposity, especially instinctive fat and truncal fat, to a great extent because of gentle energy shortages. It is through this decrease in adiposity that patients may encounter enhancements in their leptin/adiponectin levels and affectability, prompting improved hunger control and lower levels of constant aggravation hence improving a few danger factors for type 2 diabetes.

2.4 Intermittent Fasting and Insulin Sensitivity

Insulin assumes a critical part in glucose homeostasis because of its impact in advancing the capacity and use of glucose. Notwithstanding, the impacts of insulin are not restricted to glucose homeostasis. Insulin likewise assumes a part in the incitement of DNA combination, RNA amalgamation, cell development and separation, amino corrosive convergence, protein union, restraint of protein debasement, and above all, the incitement of lipogenesis and hindrance of lipolysis.

It is the advancement of insulin obstruction, which is characterized as the need of higher coursing insulin levels to create a glucose bringing down reaction that is believed to be liable for the improvement of type 2 diabetes. To advance guideline of glucose homeostasis, insulin works essentially on receptors in skeletal muscle, liver, and white fat tissue. To put it plainly, there are a few proposed components in regards to the advancement of insulin obstruction. One of the more unmistakable speculations portrays the relationship of expanded adiposity and the resulting constant aggravation that prompts the improvement of insulin opposition in tissues.

Intermittent fasting, as depicted already, may decrease adiposity and in this way insulin obstruction by means of decrease of caloric admission just as because of metabolic reconstructing. What's more, energy/supplement consumption (like that accomplished through decreased caloric admission) has been appeared to advance better maturing and decrease in constant sickness through expanded enactment of AMP initiated protein kinase (AMPK). AMPK reacts to both to expanded AMP/ADP: ATP proportions just as to endocrine signs of yearning and satiety. The part of AMPK at a biochemical level is outside of the extent of this audit, anyway actuation of AMPK through a low energy state has been appeared to start physiologic reactions that advance sound maturing. Expanded degrees of insulin, regardless of whether through expanded energy admission or insulin obstruction, prompts the initiation of downstream middle people that at last restrain AMPK. The job of AMPK in improved insulin affectability is most apparent through the beneficial outcomes of the normally endorsed biguanide, metformin. Metformin is known to advance the enactment of AMPK, and has been demonstrated to be powerful in the therapy of type 2 diabetes just as in the alleviation of various persistent infection states. In principle, diminished energy admission, for example, that is accomplished through intermittent fasting, will prompt delayed diminished degrees of insulin creation and expanded degrees of AMPK, which probably assumes a part in the upgrades in insulin affectability and glucose homeostasis.

2.5 Intermittent fasting Role in the Treatment of Type 2 Diabetes

A few investigations have shown guarantee for the utilization of intermittent fasting conventions as a likely treatment for diabetes. Tables 1 and 2 outline the discoveries of a few late examinations with respect to intermittent fasting and its impact on measures including body weight, fasting glucose, fasting insulin, adiponectin, and leptin. The consideration/rejection rules can be found in the advantageous record. In a methodical survey and Meta examination that included investigations assessing patients both with and without pre diabetes (diabetic patients were barred), it was discovered that of 8 examinations looking at the impacts of an intermittent fasting diet to a benchmark group, BMI diminished. Moreover, of 8 examinations contrasting intermittent fasting with a benchmark group in the assessment of glycemic control, it was tracked down that the intermittent fasting bunch had huge decreases in fasting glucose levels. Finally, when contrasting leptin and adiponectin levels between the intermittent fasting subjects and the control subjects in all examinations, the commentators discovered expanded adiponectin levels and diminished leptin. Followed three patients with type 2 diabetes more than a while subsequent to starting intermittent fasting routine comprising of hours diets each week. Throughout the span of the investigation, all patients had huge decreases in HbA1C, weight reduction, and the entirety of the patients had the option to stop their insulin treatment inside multi month. Curiously, the three patients for this situation arrangement all detailed enduring fasting quite well, and no tolerant halted the intercession anytime out of decision. This proposes that intermittent fasting may not exclusively be effective as a no restorative treatment choice for patients with type 2 diabetes, yet upholds the idea that this intercession is average also. Played out a clinical preliminary in which grownups with type 2 diabetes were isolated into two gatherings, one discontinuous energy limitation and ordinary eating routine each and every other day) and a constant energy limitation bunch. After whole year of mediation, the two gatherings showed comparable decreases in HbA1C levels and more noteworthy decreases in weight in the discontinuous energy limitation bunch. At long last, a comparative clinical preliminary analyzed another day fasting routine (25% of energy needs on fasting days, 125% of energy needs on no fasting days) to persistent energy limitation (75% of energy needs every day) and a benchmark group of stout, .no diabetic patients. Over an intercession time of a year, there were comparative decreases in body weight, BMI, and fat mass between the other day fasting and constant energy limitation gatherings, anyway there were critical decreases in fasting insulin levels and homeostatic model evaluation of insulin obstruction levels in the other day fasting bunch. HOMA is a marker used to gauge levels of insulin obstruction.

2.6 Recommendations for prescribing intermittent fasting in practice

While substitute day fasting and occasional fasting have exhibited viability in improving metabolic danger factors, it could be hard to persuade patients to surrender or seriously limit calories for a whole one day period. In America, we regularly eat 3 suppers each day notwithstanding successive nibbling. Besides, in American culture most friendly commitment include food. Requesting that patients kill these encounters from their everyday lives may get troublesome, and in this way obstruct patient consistence. At last, patients changing to intermittent fasting routine may at first experience indications like appetite and crabbiness, albeit these side effects frequently scatter inside the first one month. In this manner, it would be more suitable to slowly present intermittent fasting as time confined taking care of. For instance, clinicians may initially prescribe that patients confine their admission to a day by day twelve hours period, ordinarily a short term quick. As patients become more OK with this example of eating, the taking care of window can be limited further. This permits the patient some every day adaptability in picking when to devour calories, accordingly improving the probability of consistence. In conclusion, patients who have gotten adjusted to time limited taking care of may decide to change to substitute day or intermittent fasting with the management and direction of an enlisted dietician. See Fig. 5 for an itemized illustration of an intermittent fasting solution.

2.7 Considerations while prescribing intermittent fasting in practice
While thinking about the utilization of fasting in patients with diabetes, various focuses ought to be gauged. In the first place, it is critical to talk about potential dangers related with fasting. Patients taking insulin or sulfonylurea meds ought to be firmly checked by their medical services supplier to forestall hypoglycemic occasions. Since considers are showing a diminished requirement for insulin in patients who follow intermittent fasting conventions, blood glucose levels and drug titration ought to be noticed intently by the doctor. Doctors should help patients make fitting acclimations to their prescriptions, particularly on long

stretches of fasting. Doctors may decide to have patients keep day by day glucose and weight logs and send them week after week or fortnightly by means of electronic message to help suppliers in medicine titration after some time. Of note, while the objective of adjusting this example of eating is to lessen or dispense with the requirement for prescriptions, including insulin, there are circumstances in which insulin might be important, like extreme hyperglycemia. Inability to do so may bring about huge outcomes, for example, the advancement of hyperosmolar hyperglycemic condition. Extra concerns, albeit improbable, incorporate nutrient and mineral inadequacies and protein hunger. Patients ought to be instructed with respect to the significance of burning through supplement rich dinners and sufficient protein consumption during taking care of periods. Besides, it could be imperative to consider nutrient or mineral supplementation relying upon the patient's dietary practices and the ideal length of a fasting routine. Patients ought to likewise be guided on the requirement for satisfactory hydration during times of fasting, as they will be needed to supplant liquids that may typically be devoured through food notwithstanding normal every day prerequisites. As numerous doctors may not be prepared broadly in dietary sciences, and further, might not have the opportunity to follow day by day with patients to guarantee suitable healthful admission, discussion with an enrolled dietitian is energetically suggested. In conclusion, it is imperative to consider populaces in whom fasting may not be fitting. These incorporate pregnant/lactating ladies, grownups of cutting edge age, people with immunodeficiency, and people with hypoglycemic occasions, and patients who experience the ill effects of dietary problems.

2.8 Future research and Limitations

This audit is certifiably not a deliberate survey and as such does not have the ability to sum up all path with factual importance. Having said that, we featured the exploration that has been done in people and introduced proof that intermittent fasting improves insulin affectability, likely through a mix of weight reduction and "metabolic reinventing". There is a lot of exploration that has been done on the impacts of intermittent fasting concerning enhancements in body arrangement and metabolic wellbeing, anyway a lion's share of the information to date has come from creature contemplates, which were excluded from this survey. Despite the fact that there are various case reports showing critical upgrades in diabetic patients' glucose control, large numbers of the randomized controlled preliminaries neglect to incorporate patients with diabetes. This is a territory where further examination is required, as the current preliminaries (and case reports) remembered for this audit that have been done on diabetic patients have shown guarantee in improving metabolic wellbeing with almost no antagonistic impacts. Most patients doing some type of intermittent fasting experience gentle energy deficiencies and weight reduction that may not be suitable for all patients. Thusly, there should be more investigation into outlining the metabolic upgrades of intermittent fasting from weight reduction.

Type 2 diabetes distresses 34.2 million individuals in the United States, and is related with huge horribleness and mortality. Despite the fact that diabetes is portrayed as a turmoil of insulin obstruction, a lion's share of the drug medicines for this illness advance expansions in insulin levels to accomplish better glycemic control. This prompts various issues including weight acquire, demolished insulin opposition, expanded degrees of leptin, and diminished degrees of adiponectin. Intermittent fasting has become an inexorably known dietary practice for the improvement of body structure and metabolic wellbeing. It likewise has shown guarantee in the treatment of type 2 diabetes. This might be because of its consequences for weight reduction, as well as diminishing insulin opposition and an ideal change in the degrees of leptin and adiponectin. Patients may move toward their doctors with questions in regards to the execution of intermittent fasting. Also, doctors ought to know about the advantages of this dietary practice as a treatment for type 2 diabetes with the goal that they might have the option to help patients utilize this to battle the movement of their sickness.

2.9 Intermittent Fasting in Diabetes Mellitus Patients: Clinical Management

Intermittent fasting is expanding in notoriety as a methods for getting in shape and controlling persistent disease. Patients with diabetes mellitus, the two kinds 1 and 2, include about 10% of the populace in the United States and would probably be pulled in to follow one of the numerous strategies for intermittent fasting. Studies on the security and advantages of intermittent fasting with diabetes are exceptionally restricted however, and wellbeing suggestions shockingly today emerge principally from weight reduction masters and creature contemplates. Clinical rules on the most proficient method to oversee restorative intermittent fasting in patients with diabetes are nonexistent. The proof to assemble a particularly clinical rule for individuals with a diabetes determination is practically nonexistent, with only one randomized preliminary and a few case reports. This article gives an outline of the accessible information and a survey of the exceptionally restricted relevant writing on the impacts of intermittent fasting among individuals with diabetes. It additionally assesses the known wellbeing and viability issues encompassing medicines for diabetes in the fasting state. In light of those restricted information and an information on accepted procedures, this paper proposes master put together rules with respect to how to deal with a patient with either type 1 or 2 diabetes who is keen on intermittent fasting. The security of each significant drug treatment during a fasting period is thought of. At the point when done under the oversight of the patient's medical services supplier, and with fitting individual glucose observing, intermittent fasting can be securely embraced in patients with diabetes.

The term intermittent fasting implies diminished caloric admission on a discontinuous premise. This can differ from a few hours during the day to a total 24 h period. It tends to be accomplished for strict reasons, for example, during Ramadan or Yom Kippur, or for wellbeing reasons, including weight reduction. In this article, we will address just non strict intermittent fasting directed for wellbeing purposes and will audit the advantages, either potential or demonstrated, just as security worries in patients with diabetes mellitus, the two kinds 1 and 2. Articles have been composed on the most proficient method to oversee strict fasting and the per user inspired by this subject is alluded to these articles

The term intermittent fasting, when utilized for wellbeing reasons or weight reduction, has been utilized to portray different sorts of caloric limitation. A few creators use it when a patient retains caloric admission for a few sequential hours during the day (regularly 16 h with all energy consumption during the other 8 h of the day), others for an entire day more than once per week, and others three or four days of the week. A few conventions permit protein consumption yet no carbs and still name it intermittent fasting. Others permit carbs or large scale/miniature supplements up to a furthest reaches that will in any case advance ketosis and, despite the fact that it is just a low calorie diet, because of the prevalence of fasting this has been named an eating regimen that imitates fasting. In all cases, no caloric liquid admission is allowed (which is one of the fundamental contrasts when contrasted with strict fasting) and thusly essentially decreases the danger of drying out and hypotension, a conspicuous thought in strict fasting.

2.9.1 How it Work?
Most investigations of intermittent fasting have zeroed in on weight reduction as the essential objective. Those

investigations were led under the idea that the essential medical advantage of intermittent fasting emerges from weight reduction. Along these lines, the time confined taking care of, substitute day fasting, and 5:2 eating routine regimens are not planned to be ketotic, however to essentially actuate upgrades in wellbeing through the average components related with weight reduction. For a more intensive audit of human investigations of the impact of intermittent fasting on changes in weight.

While ketosis is neither an objective nor an assumption for those supper timing plans, some fasting regimens may accomplish ketosis. Somebody have utilized the expression "metabolic switch" to portray "the body's special shift from use of glucose from glycogenolysis to unsaturated fats and unsaturated fat inferred ketones". They bring up that "ketones are the favored fuel for both the cerebrum and body during times of fasting and expanded exercise".

The metabolic switch happens when glycogen stores in the liver are exhausted, for the most part 12 h after the suspension of food admission, and fat tissue lipolysis increments to create more unsaturated fats and glycerol. The free unsaturated fats are shipped to the liver where they are oxidized to beta hydroxybutyrate and acetoacetate. They are changed over to energy through beta oxidation. By and large, this cycle includes expanded coursing unsaturated fats and different changes identified with glucose and unsaturated fat digestion, whose changes were as of late detailed among people during water just fasting.

Peroxisome proliferator initiated receptor alpha incites the statement of qualities that intervene unsaturated fat oxidation in muscle cells. Curiously, insulin opposition delays the time it takes to flip the metabolic switch and along these lines among individuals with diabetes it might take more time to start utilizing unsaturated fats for energy. The entirety of the ramifications of this distinction are not seen yet conceivably have suggestions for the board of individuals with diabetes who participate in intermittent fasting, however this requires examination in individuals with diabetes.

In those regimens that don't include genuine fasting, the "metabolic switch" component would not draw in and apparently the system of activity is essentially diminished caloric admission. Other expected instruments of medical advantages from fasting are under examination presently. These remember the expected effect of intermittent fasting for aggravation, receptive oxygen species, circulatory strain, and cholesterol levels, a portion of whose changes may happen just because of weight reduction yet that may conceivably likewise be affected through instruments that are free of weight change. They likewise may remember an effect for the human micro biome, the human development chemical/insulin like development factor 1 pivot, mitochondriogenesis, invulnerable framework productivity, and autophagy. Autophagy directs the amino corrosive inventory, and this was as of late answered to be controlled in explicit examples during water just fasting in people. Beforehand, an example of expanded oxygen helping limit through higher erythrocyte tally and hemoglobin levels during water just fasting was accounted for that may improve metabolic working or abatement insulin obstruction. Different systems may likewise exist that are simply starting to be investigated. Further assessment of the components of conceivable wellbeing impacts of intermittent fasting in people is expected to completely comprehend the effect that it has on human wellbeing.

2.9.2 Benefits of Clinical Management

Insulin obstruction, the most unmistakable element of type 2 diabetes, has for some time been known to improve with caloric limitation. After a time of fasting, insulin affectability rises and insulin levels fall. These outcome in improved fasting and postprandial glucose levels. Furthermore, as insulin incites fat tissue development, there is less inclination to weight acquire and conceivably even weight reduction.

Intermittent fasting would thus be able to be required to impact weight reduction, particularly when it is led regularly. From the get go in the investigation of fasting's wellbeing impacts it was guessed that fasting could improve a portion of the significant bothersome impacts of weight reduction slims down. Intermittent fasting has now been appeared, in any case, in different little and momentary investigations to be correspondingly powerful as every day calorie limitation in delivering weight reduction. Along these lines, when done as often as sufficiently possible, fasting can be one alternative for sound weight reduction, however the best proof shows that fasting is certifiably not an unrivaled weight reduction technique.

Insulin obstruction is related with an expanded fiery state including raised C-responsive protein, diminished adiponectin, lower low thickness lipoprotein (LDL) molecule size, and other metabolic elements that all add to or are related with atherosclerosis and improvement of coronary course infection.

Besides, insulin is referred to be both atherogenic just as increment the danger of liquid maintenance and congestive cardiovascular breakdown. Subsequently, decreasing insulin levels through intermittent fasting would have the potential for diminishing major antagonistic cardiovascular occasions. Such decrease in insulin might be attainable. Written about three patients who had the option to suspend insulin treatment 5–18 days in the wake of starting intermittent fasting, during which they had supper however skipped breakfast and lunch on either substitute days or 3 days out of every week. Further examination of this speculation in bigger populaces is required, yet this finding is an enticing and possibly outlook changing outcome in the event that it tends to be securely and dependably rehashed in enormous populaces.

Intermittent fasting and calorie limitation have been appeared to improve different metabolic and fiery pathways. Included are expanded warmth stun protein, advancing cell autophagy, diminishing progressed glycation final results, expanded adiponectin, and diminished aggravation cytokines. Every one of these impacts bring about diminished vascular brokenness and would consequently be required to improve cardiovascular danger as well as mortality. Regardless of whether indeed the progressions because of fasting are critical and supported enough to do so stays to be demonstrated.

While there are no imminent clinical preliminaries of cardiovascular advantages from intermittent fasting (i.e., its impacts on clinical major unfriendly cardiovascular occasions), observational populace examines have shown cardiovascular and metabolic advantages a lower hazard of coronary course illness and lower hazard of diabetes from just one day out of each long stretch of energy limitation through fasting (rehearsed over a time of many years). One planned clinical preliminary did as of late report an impact of intermittent fasting on the control of hemoglobin A1C. Among a populace of 97 individuals with type 2 diabetes mellitus (40 of the 137 took a crack at the preliminary pulled out right on time), hemoglobin A1C decrease because of intermittent fasting was non subpar compared to persistent energy limitation. Sadly, weight reduction in that preliminary was not diverse in the fasting arm contrasted with caloric limitation, and other metabolic measures were not extraordinary. Generally, audits of the proof show that deficient human information exist as of now to suggest the utilization of intermittent fasting or low calorie diets to forestall diabetes or, among individuals with diabetes, to forestall its sequel.

2.9.3 Risk Factors

The most impending danger with intermittent fasting is the potential for hypoglycemia in patients who are on ant diabetic drugs that are related with hypoglycemia, explicitly insulin (both prandial and basal) and sulfonylureas (counting the short acting meglitinides). Any remaining ant diabetic prescriptions when utilized either as mono therapy or in mix treatment without insulin or sulfonylureas are infrequently, however not never, related with hypoglycemia, and the danger is in this way significantly less however still a thought.

With long haul intermittent fasting, one requirements to likewise be worried about protein ailing health if patients are not conscious to keep up satisfactory protein admission on those occasions when they are eating. Nutrient and mineral lack of healthy sustenance could likewise happen and, contingent upon how long seven days the patient is fasting and what they are eating when they do eat, might require taking nutrient as well as mineral enhancements.

Different dangers incorporate an assortment of potential damages identified with deficient energy admission and some because of lack of hydration. These incorporate wellbeing occasions that may happen among any individual who takes part in intermittent fasting, whether or not they have diabetes. Such unfavorable occasions may incorporate discombobulating, queasiness, a sleeping disorder, syncope, falls, headache migraine, shortcoming that limits day by day exercises, and exorbitant cravings for food. The presence of a constant illness, including diabetes, may expand the danger of encountering a significant number of these antagonistic occasions, as may different sicknesses including coronary vein infection, shaky angina, cardiovascular breakdown, atrial fibrillation, earlier myocardial dead tissue, earlier stroke or transient ischemic assault, most malignant growths, ongoing obstructive aspiratory infection, pneumonic embolism, asthma, fringe vascular thromboembolism, persistent kidney infection, and possibly different conditions. For individuals with these persistent sicknesses, little is thought about the reaction to fasting, in this way it isn't really that they ought not to take part in fasting, however that how their dangers because of fasting are changed is dubious and expect studies to be led in these populaces where raised wellbeing hazards exist. Positively, presenting such people to genuine unfriendly occasions like new myocardial dead tissue, stroke, or passing is unjustifiable and alert is the key as of now given the absence of proof in these populaces.

For conditions where drying out is a danger, like stroke, consolation to hydrate well during any fasting routine is suggested. Drinking water, including to supplant liquids that regularly would be devoured in food sources, is a significant thought for individuals of any age who are partaking in intermittent fasting.

Moreover, a few populaces have exceptional dangers and ought to be discouraged from taking part in intermittent fasting, particularly on the off chance that they have diabetes. This incorporates pregnant and lactating ladies, small kids, grownups of cutting edge age, and more established grownups who are delicate. People with immune deficiencies, including the individuals who have had a strong organ relocate and are on clinical immunosuppression, ought to likewise shun fasting. Individuals with dietary issues and those with dementia have special difficulties that will probably be exacerbated by purposely captivating in fasting, subsequently they ought not to follow intermittent fasting regimens. Patients who have a background marked by awful mind injury or post concussive condition may likewise be at higher danger of antagonistic occasions, and their necessities ought to be viewed as cautiously dependent upon the situation before starting a fasting routine.

2.9.4 Management
Patients with diabetes who are keen on intermittent fasting ought to be urged to take part in fasting with direction from a medical services professional, including doctors, nurture experts, doctors' aides, ensured diabetes teachers, or enlisted dietitians. Explicit consideration ought to be paid to three contemplations: prescription change, recurrence of glucose checking, and liquid admission. The majority of these proposals depend on the clinical experience of the creators when there is no free writing, while a portion of the suggestions depend on distributed methodologies in investigations of intermittent fasting among individuals with diabetes.

2.9.5 Glucose Monitoring
Except if the patient is utilizing a sulfonylurea or insulin, the danger of hypoglycemia is low and no extra glucose

checking would be regularly suggested during fasting. The patient ought to, nonetheless, be helped about the side effects to remember hypoglycemia and ought to be urged to check their blood glucose if any of the indications do create. A few patients will create manifestations reminiscent of hypoglycemia even with a blood glucose over 70 mg/dL, hence alert is demonstrated in the way to deal with their reaction to indications related to glucose checking.

In patients on a sulfonylurea or insulin (either alone or in mix with some other ant diabetic medicine), the danger of hypoglycemia is huge, and the patient ought to be urged to accomplish more regular blood glucose testing, particularly when initially beginning with intermittent fasting. Contingent upon the danger of hypoglycemia as surveyed by the expert, the testing could be as frequently as at regular intervals in the patient on insulin or like clockwork on sulfonylureas. On the off chance that the fasting is a 24 h or longer quick, particularly a water just quick, explicit thoughtfulness regarding the following daytime's fasting blood glucose perusing ought to be made.

Patients on insulin who will embrace intermittent fasting may be urged to utilize individual ceaseless glucose observing frameworks. On account of the framework, this would consider a hypoglycemia alert. With the Freestyle framework, while there is no hypoglycemia ready, continuous testing should be possible without extra cost or distress. The danger of hypoglycemia with intermittent fasting while at the same time utilizing insulin can't be over underscored and may even increment if the patient is effective in getting more fit because of the discontinuous quick. While depending on finger stick glucose testing might be satisfactory, having a nonstop glucose observing framework would by and large urge the patient to accomplish more regular glucose testing and manage the cost of the extra security that accompanies more continuous testing.

2.9.6 Intake of Fluids

While patients will drink non caloric fluids during intermittent fasting, patients may not understand that except if they drink extra fluids, they are really decreasing their complete liquid admission because of diminished admission of food sources like soups, yogurt, or melons. For this situation, the danger of parchedness and hypotension increments. The patient may then have to decrease or retain their admission of diuretics, SGLT-2 inhibitors, or hostile to hypertensive drugs on the times of fasting.

Conclusion

Intermittent fasting, when embraced for wellbeing reasons in patients with diabetes mellitus, the two kinds 1 and 2, has been appeared in a couple of little human examinations to prompt weight reduction and diminish insulin necessities. While these discoveries are energizing and have caught the creative mind of numerous individuals, an astute way to deal with executing fasting regimens and utilizing them in the long haul among this particular populace is required. A significant part of the promotion encompassing fasting emerges from creature examines, which just propose what human exploration ought to be directed; execution of human intercessions ought not to be founded on creature research.

Long haul advantages of fasting, including cardiovascular danger decrease, stay to be completely considered and clarified, particularly in people. Clinicians should temper the eagerness for fasting with the truth that the advantages and dangers in people remain to a great extent neglected and the advantages may require a long time to years to show up or be completely figured it out. Great proof from epidemiologic investigations, pilot interventional preliminaries, and a couple of randomized preliminaries recommends that the advantages of fasting exceed the likely damages in the normal person. Individuals with diabetes, be that as it may, are not the normal individual, and their own necessities require more cautious thought toward the start of and during the utilization of a fasting routine. With legitimate drug change and observing of blood glucose levels however, intermittent fasting can be supported and securely executed among individuals with diabetes.

CPSIA information can be obtained
at www.ICGtesting.com
Printed in the USA
BVHW052027080521
606756BV00004B/958

9 781802 263374